HEALING H. PYLORI HANDBOOK

THE EFFECTIVE WAYS OF HEALING H. PYLORI

DR. MATT NORMAN

Table of Contents

CHAPTER ONE

Which Drug Is Most Effective Against H. pylori?

Briefly, H. pylori is a bacterium that can lead to stomach ulcers and other health issues.

GORD is an acronym for gastroesophageal reflux disease, which is an infection of the stomach caused by the bacteria Helicobacter pylori (H. pylori). Probiotics, according to a study published in 2020, can keep the bad bacteria in your gut in check while keeping the good bacteria in your gut in healthy numbers. Antibiotics for H. pylori work better when combined with probiotics, which prevent the growth of harmful bacteria while killing off the good.

Beneficial microorganisms can be replenished with the help of probiotics. You may find yourself less susceptible to yeast infections as a result. Lactobacillus acidophilus is the best probiotic strain.

H. pylori is responsible for up to 95% of duodenal and peptic ulcer cases in developing countries, but only 30% to 50% in developed nations. It may take time for symptoms of H. pylori infection to present themselves. Many people who are infected with H. pylori are clueless as to the fact that they have the disease. The digestive system may also be affected, with symptoms including:

• severe stomach pain

gas pains

Feeling sick

a complete lack of hunger

Urinary urgency or frequency

• unexplained weight loss

Gastrocnemius cancer

Some people, for instance, may experience severe negative reactions to antibiotics. Possible negative reactions to this drug include feeling sick, having diarrhea, and losing your appetite.

Some patients may be harder to treat with conventional methods due to antibiotic resistance. This has led to a rise in the popularity of natural treatments for H. pylori. This is something you can use in conjunction with your doctor-prescribed medical care. They can be used independently in some situations.

How effective are natural remedies for H. pylori?

Both in vitro and in vivo research has been conducted on natural treatments for H. pylori. For the most part, treatment was successful in lowering but not completely eliminating the number of bacteria in the stomach.

Talk to your doctor before starting any alternative treatment. The recommended treatment for H. pylori should not be substituted with natural remedies.

With your doctor's blessing, you can use complementary therapies like natural remedies. This may improve the efficiency of conventional drugs.

Probiotics

When taken regularly, probiotics support a digestive system with a favorable ratio of good bacteria to harmful pathogens. A study scheduled for completion in 2020 suggests that taking probiotics either before or after conventional H. pylori treatment may increase eradication success.

Probiotics are a great way to restore the good bacteria in your stomach after taking antibiotics. You may find yourself less susceptible to yeast infections as a result. The best bacteria, according to the studies, is lactobacillus acidophilus.

Pros:

boosts the population of good bacteria in the gut

can aid in the reduction of belly fat.

Cons:

has the potential to trigger stomach and bowel problems

This • could cause some unpleasant side effects, like headaches.

Green-tea-based tea

In a study from 2020, researchers found that using a mouthwash containing an extract of green tea reduced the growth of Helicobacter bacteria. Lots of different green teas are available here.

Pros:

owing to its high polyphenol content, it is able to mitigate inflammation.

Fat loss: • Possible temporary boost

Cons:

Green tea contains caffeine, so moderation is recommended.

Honey

Honey has anti-H. pylori properties that have recently been discovered. Extensive research supports these conclusions. To date, studies have not shown that honey can kill the bacteria outright, but it can slow their growth. Incorporating honey into current treatments has the potential to speed up the recovery process. Raw honey and Manuka honey, in particular, may have the strongest antibacterial properties.

Pros:

A healthier heart might be a possible benefit.

helpful in preventing cell damage; rich in antioxidants

Cons:

weight gain due to sugar characterized by a high sugar content

Olive oil, in other words.

Olive oil's antimicrobial properties may make it useful

for warding off H. pylori infection. Olive oil is a healthy alternative that can be used in cooking and salad dressings.

Pros:

effects on inflammation reduction

Improved bone and heart health are a possible benefit.

Cons:

High in calories

Potential for allergic reactions

Origin of licorice.

Licorice root is a safe and effective treatment for stomach ulcers. Another target worth considering is H. pylori. A review conducted in 2020 discovered that licorice root had an antibacterial effect, which increased the rate at which bacteria were eliminated. It appears to aid in preventing H. pylori from adhering to cell walls, in addition to promoting ulcer healing. Some medications may not work as well if taken with licorice root, which can be bought online.

Check with your medical professional before adding licorice root to your treatment regimen.

Pros:

There's some evidence that it could help with stomach pain and indigestion.

- may be useful for treating stomach ulcers

Cons:

It is known to interact with a wide variety of drugs, including nonsteroidal anti-inflammatory drugs (NSAIDs), blood thinners, statins, and diuretics.

may not be the most effective tactic in the long run. (Long-term or excessive licorice root use can lead to glycopyrrhizin accumulation in the body.)

broccoli sprouts

It has been proposed that the compound sulforaphane, which is found in broccoli sprouts, could be used to treat H. pylori infection. Broccoli sprouts' anti-inflammatory and digestive-health-boosting antioxidant properties are well-documented.

That could mean less bacterial colonization and the problems that come with it.

For those struggling with type 2 diabetes, taking a supplement of powdered broccoli sprouts has been shown to be an effective way to fight H. pylori. In addition, factors associated with cardiovascular risk were lowered. Two studies conducted in 2020 and 2021, however, suggest that sulforaphane may not be as effective as previously thought at eliminating or reducing H. pylori, especially in cases of severe infections.

Pros:

This approach has the potential to reduce inflammation and enhance digestive health.

The benefits to cardiovascular health are:

Cons:

There is a high risk of bacterial contamination, so make sure you wash your hands thoroughly before eating.

• Your thyroid's ability to work might be impacted by your habit of overeating.

Additional studies are required to confirm that H. pylori treatments are effective.

Phototherapy

LED blue light therapy may be useful for treating H. pylori that is resistant to antibiotics. Phototherapy, which makes use of ultraviolet light, is effective against the stomach bacterium H. pylori. By reducing tissue damage and H. pylori activity, blue LED endoscopy improved the efficacy of curcumin therapy. Intestinal phototherapy is thought to be safe by some researchers. This could be useful in situations where antibiotics aren't feasible.

Pros:

• this is helpful if you're trying to avoid antibiotics

Cons:

As you can see, this is a stopgap measure at best. (The bacteria will repopulate a few days after phototherapy.)

Curcumin

Curcumin, found in turmeric, is the active ingredient. Curcumin has strong anti-inflammatory and anti-oxidant properties.

A recent study found that curcumin mitigated inflammation and stopped H. pylori from damaging gastric cells. Damaged gastric tissue can recover more rapidly as a result of the enhanced blood supply. Furthermore, it enhanced gut-brain communication, which in turn improved the body's immune response.

Due to curcumin's anti-inflammatory and antibacterial properties, the authors conclude that taking it in conjunction with triple therapy is beneficial.

Treatments used historically for H. pylori

Two antibiotics and an acid-reducing drug are typically used to treat H. pylori. Triple therapy is so named because it consists of three different treatments.

If you cannot take the antibiotics prescribed, you may be prescribed alternative medications. The H. pylori bacteria must be reduced by at least 90% for treatment to be effective.

In some cases, treatment for an H. pylori-related ulcer can take longer than two weeks. Using a combination of two antibiotics is preferable to using just one, as this helps to slow the development of antibiotic resistance. The antibiotics used to combat H. pylori include:

1. amoxicillin

A. Tetracycline

* Metronidazole

* Clarithromycin

Stomach acid-reducing drugs help the body heal. To name a few of them:

Omeprazole (Prilosec) and lansoprazole (Prevacid) are two drugs used to treat acid reflux and peptic ulcers.

Histamine blockers that work by preventing the production of stomach acid include cimetidine (Tagamet).

Bismuth subsalicylate, the active ingredient in Pepto-Bismol,

coats and protects your stomach
lining.

CHAPTER TWO

People can carry the bacteria for decades, even a lifetime, without ever experiencing any ill effects. Neglecting to treat chronic stomach inflammation can have serious consequences. Diseases like stomach cancer and stomach ulcers that cause bleeding are examples. H. pylori infection has been associated with a subset of stomach cancers.

High rates of H. pylori eradication are seen when antibiotic treatment that has been approved by the FDA is used. The highest incidence is seen when antibiotics are combined with an acid neutralizer. There is potential for natural therapies to enhance the healing process.

Seize the moment and make the most of your current circumstances.

In the United States, testing for H. pylori is uncommon outside of the context of diagnosing symptoms. If you're experiencing any of these signs, please contact your doctor immediately. H. pylori infection shares symptoms with gastroesophageal reflux disease. It is essential that you get the right treatment based on an accurate diagnosis.

When other causes cannot be ruled out, a colonoscopy or endoscopy may be required.

If H. pylori is detected, treatment should begin immediately. Natural remedies are safe to use, but there is no proof that they can eradicate the infection entirely. Do not use them in place of conventional treatments without first consulting with your doctor.

a millisecond's worth of time,
divided by zero

Absolutely no space is involved.

CHAPTER THREE

Instructions for Future
Infection Prevention

The etiology of H. pylori is unknown. The Centers for Disease Control and Prevention (CDC) has not released any official recommendations for avoiding this. It is recommended that you cook your food thoroughly and wash your hands frequently. If H. pylori is confirmed, see your doctor regularly and finish the prescribed treatment.

The most frequently asked questions are:

False, H. pylori can be gotten rid of without the use of antibiotics.

Following your doctor's instructions for taking antibiotics is essential if you want to completely eradicate H. pylori from your system.

To eliminate H. pylori with lemon water, or not to worry?

Lemon water is not effective against H. pylori. Its acidity could make your symptoms worse.

Do you think ginger helps with H. pylori?

As much as ginger may help with gastrointestinal distress, it cannot completely eliminate H. pylori from the stomach.

What are the most effective methods for treating H. pylori using only natural ingredients?

The bacterium Helicobacter pylori thrives in the acidic environment of an infected stomach (H. pylori). These microbes are a known contributor to peptic and duodenal ulcers. Natural remedies might not be able to completely get rid of the bacteria, but they could keep it to a manageable level.

Inflammation of the stomach caused by H. pylori can progress to gastritis, ulcers, and even stomach cancer. H. pylori infections typically call for triple therapy, consisting of two antibiotics and a proton pump inhibitor.

Antibiotics may cause side effects in some people. Natural remedies may be able to mitigate these negative effects, as well as protect the stomach, aid in infection prevention, and improve general health.

Since H. pylori is notoriously difficult to get rid of, some patients may opt to combine conventional treatment with natural remedies.

CHAPTER FOUR

Removing H. pylori through all-natural means is possible.

H. pylori infection treatments that are non-invasive to the body have been the subject of extensive scientific inquiry. Eight all-natural remedies are listed below.

Honey, to begin with.

Some people have found success using natural remedies to treat their H. pylori infections.

Honey's antibacterial properties have made it a popular remedy since ancient times.

In one study, Manuka honey was found to inhibit the proliferation of human gastric epithelial cells.

Honey has been shown to have anti-pylori properties in some studies, but more are needed to determine its efficacy as a complementary or alternative treatment.

Aloe vera is a type of plant.

Aloe vera has been used to treat a wide variety of conditions, including:

• bowel obstruction

The Detox Process

Wellness in regards to one's diet

Regeneration of damaged tissue

The gel extracted from the inner leaves of an aloe vera plant was effective at inhibiting the growth of and killing drug-resistant H. pylori strains in laboratory tests.

This study suggests that aloe vera, when used in conjunction with antibiotics, can help treat H. pylori infection.

broccoli sprouts

Broccoli sprouts contain a compound called sulforaphane, which has been shown to be effective against H. pylori.

In vitro, in vivo, and in human studies, sulforaphane has been shown to inhibit the growth of H. pylori bacteria. In mice infected with Helicobacter pylori, Broccoli sprouts also decreased gastric inflammation.

There are 4 fluid ounces in a glass of milk.

Inhibition of Helicobacter pylori growth by the glycoprotein lactoferrin has been demonstrated. This glycoprotein is present in both human and cow milk. There were no lingering symptoms of H. pylori after treatment with antibiotics and lactoferrin from cow's milk in a study of 150 patients.

Also, melanoidin appears to have antibacterial effects against the bacterium H. pylori. Melanoidin is a compound found in fruits and vegetables that is formed when the lactose and casein in milk and dairy products react. It has been shown that melanoidin can prevent H. pylori colonization in both mice and humans.

Fifth, lemongrass's volatile oil

Humans should avoid ingesting essential oils. Alternatively, they can use aromatherapy to benefit from the scents by inhaling them. The growth of H. pylori can be slowed by using lemongrass essential oil, and this effect has been observed in both humans and animals.

The colonization of the stomachs of mice treated with lemongrass oil was significantly lower than that of mice not treated with oil.

GREEN TEA!

Green tea's widespread popularity can be attributed to its many positive health effects. In addition to being a great source of antioxidants, it is also rich in nutrients and a good source of vitamins and minerals.

In an animal study, the number of bacteria and the severity of inflammation caused by H. pylori were both reduced by green tea. The mice that were given green tea before infection, however, fared much better.

Probiotics are beneficial bacteria that can help the body.

According to the Food and Agriculture Organization, probiotics are beneficial microorganisms that can be consumed by humans. Treatment of H. pylori with probiotics is gaining popularity.

There is a wide range of probiotic supplements available. Dairy bacteria and those found in other fermented foods are frequently used to treat and prevent stomach ailments.

Science has proven that Bifidobacterium can kill H. pylori by interfering with the bacterium's ability to adhere to the stomach lining.

8. light therapy

Studies have shown that the H. pylori bacteria are vulnerable to ultraviolet light. During phototherapy, an ultraviolet light source shines on the entire stomach.

Stomach bacteria can be drastically reduced with photosynthetic therapy. Once the lights come back on, however, the bacteria will quickly multiply and spread.

Phototherapy has the potential to be an effective treatment for H. pylori for those who cannot take antibiotics.

When is it time to see a doctor?

Nausea is a common symptom of an H. pylori infection.

This bacteria can live dormant in the body for decades without causing any harm. H. pylori testing is not commonly performed by doctors. The first step in effectively treating a condition is determining what it is.

Possible signs of an H. pylori infection include:

• abdominal pain

inner-body burns

gas pains

Feeling sick

• heartburn

a complete lack of hunger

Those who experience a change in their health should consult a doctor immediately. You shouldn't try to treat H. pylori with natural remedies instead of antibiotics unless your doctor specifically recommends it.

CHAPTER FIVE

Takeaway

H. pylori is a type of bacteria that lives in the digestive tract and is a leading cause of gastric and duodenal ulcers and bleeding.

Because the pylori bacteria have become antibiotic-resistant, traditional antibiotics are no longer effective in treating the infection.

Some natural treatments have been shown to be ineffective against H. pylori bacteria.

The best course of action when dealing with H. pylori infection is to consult a medical professional before trying any alternative remedies.

In rare cases, a drug may have an adverse reaction to a herbal supplement or vitamin. The Food and Drug Administration (FDA) in the United States does not regulate the quality or purity of supplements, so shoppers should do their research and talk to their doctor before taking any.